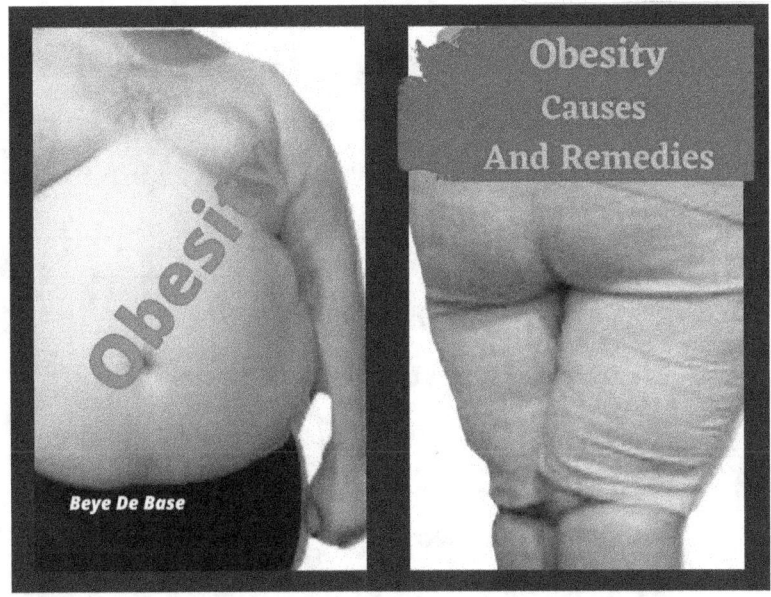

Obesity Causes And Remedies

By : Beye De Base

SUMMARY

Parents' main nightmare is the recurrent illness of their children. Millions of children die every year because of an illness that is not taken seriously from the start.

One-third of children and adolescents and 66% of the adult population are overweight or obese. If this trend continues, the life expectancy of our children will decrease, making them the first generation to live less than their parents.

You may be trying to help your child lose weight, or you may feel that your child is at risk of becoming overweight or unhealthy because of his eating and exercise habits.

Childhood illness such as obesity will be discussed in this book to help you understand the causes and cures.

• Causes Of Childhood Obesity

As a child, do you remember being given a lot of food and being told to swallow every bit of it? Have you met parents who believe that fat children make happy and healthy children? This is one of the reasons for the increase in cases of childhood obesity around the world.

• What is Obesity?

Obesity means that the body contains too much fat. To describe it scientifically, obesity is characterized by a weight measurement and a body mass index well above the norm. It results from a high caloric intake and a very low energy expenditure.

Obesity is a growing problem, not only in the U.S., but around the world. A recent study showed that in the United States alone, 65% of the population is overweight and obese. Worldwide, an estimated 300 million adults are obese. Fifteen percent of the U.S. child population has also been reported to be overweight. Worldwide, an estimated twenty-two million children aged five and under are overweight.

• What Causes Childhood Obesity?

Like any other medical condition, childhood obesity can be caused by a number of factors, most often in combination. Obesity can be either: acquired by external factors, hereditary, caused by psychological factors, or secondary to a current condition.

1. Acquired.

It can result from poor eating habits, and lack of physical activity to burn calories from previous food intake contributes to a peak in weight gain.

2. Hereditary.

Children born to obese parents are more likely to be overweight and obese themselves. This is usually due to unhealthy eating habits observed in the parents.

3. Psychological Factors.

Obesity may be secondary for children who eat too much to cope with stress and/or negative emotions such as: boredom, anger, sadness, anxiety or depression.

4. Diseases.

Various conditions such as hypothyroidism, Cushing's syndrome, depression and other neurological problems can lead to obesity and weight gain in children.

Will there be complications?

If a child continues to engage in poor eating habits and does not engage in physical activity to burn calories, childhood obesity can lead to life-threatening complications, including diabetes, high blood pressure, heart disease, sleep disorders, cancer and other health problems. Overweight children are likely to become overweight adults as well.

Most often, obese children are subject to public teasing and humiliation. To a certain extent, this even leads to harassment, violence and even discrimination from his or her family. The children then grow up with very low self-esteem and suffer from depression.

What Can We Do To Prevent Childhood Obesity?

It is never good to ignore the signs of childhood obesity. Action is needed to establish good health before your child's obesity gets worse.

Set an achievable weight loss goal. Your goals should not be overly ambitious and should allow room for normal growth and development. Start small, so as not to overwhelm or discourage your child with the changes you plan to implement.

Manage your child's diet. Keep a journal or list of the foods your child eats daily. This will help you make a more accurate assessment of your child's diet. This food journal should be as detailed as possible.

Reserve time for physical activities. Exercise is necessary for continuous weight loss. It also helps to redistribute body fat into the muscles. Again, start small so as not to discourage the child. Slowly increase the amount of time spent exercising for best results.

In conclusion, childhood obesity is a condition that is totally reversible. The best thing you can do to avoid this kind of dilemma for your child is to set a good example. Show them how good eating habits and a healthy lifestyle can help you enjoy life more. It's the best way to show them that you care about them too.

• Childhood Obesity In Our Youth

Seeing a child being abused is one of the worst things a mother can endure, so why is your child's obesity different? Childhood obesity is on the rise, as is adult obesity, so why are we all focusing on adult thinness when it should be children who are the focus of our attention? An obese child is a problem that cannot go unanswered. The child will have serious problems in his or her life if he or she does not lose this weight. He will be unhappy and unfit for the rest of his life if no one takes care of him, as he is supposed to know he is a child, it is the parents' responsibility to make sure that the child gets better!

A child is less likely to be obese due to health problems, and although genetics play a role in his or her obesity, it is the lifestyle of the family that contributes most to the disease. To be frank, most cases of childhood obesity are due to poor nutrition and lack of exercise. Although in this day and age, being overweight comes as no surprise with junk food, take-out and sweets everywhere you go and convenience, not health, is on everyone's mind! Not to mention that most kids would rather sit and watch TV or play at their consoles than go outside to play! Exercise is no longer part of children's routine, they are lucky to have two hours of exercise at school and at home; there is none. The National Food and Nutrition Survey conducted in 2000 showed that 40-69% of children were not exercising for the recommended one hour a day, and it is worrisome that this number has increased.

Childhood obesity can be sorted out if it is treated at an early age, we don't want to have to watch our children get bullied at school for being overweight, or have surgery to prevent them from eating so much. We need to show our children that they need to eat sensibly and we need to get them active. Most children copy their parents' examples, so if we have to eat fresh fruits and vegetables, there's no reason why they shouldn't do so. To help prevent childhood obesity, try to eliminate a lot of sugary foods from the home and replace them with nutritious foods like fruits and low-fat alternatives.

In addition to increased mortality, childhood obesity increases the likelihood of chronic disease and we must prevent this, we must show our children that being overweight is not the life they should lead and that parents should focus on getting their children to eat properly, otherwise obesity will lead us all to disaster.

• How to Help Your Child Fight Childhood Obesity?

Halloween, sleep parties, birthdays - sometimes it feels like childhood is a big food holiday. It's hard to deprive your child of special treats and pleasures when all his friends are having a big party.

However, this simple condition may cause more problems than you think. Treating your child from time to time may be a good thing, but giving him the opportunity to devour all the sweets and treats he wants could mean a big problem: childhood obesity.

In some cases, some people claim that genetics may play a major role in childhood obesity. This is true, but not as much as the role of parents. It is not true that genetic material causes a child to be heavy from an early age.

For most of the population, genetic material can set lower maximum values for people's weight, but people themselves set higher maximum values through their food choices. In addition, since most children cannot simply set limits and choose the foods they should eat, it is the duty of parents to set the limits.

You don't know how to do it? Here are a few tips to help you follow your child's diet and nutrition and fight childhood obesity.

- Happy Halloween!

The only holiday devoted almost entirely to the overconsumption of "sweet treats", Halloween holds an extraordinary place in hell for most parents faced with childhood obesity.

It's understandable that this is a very difficult time for your child, but you can make it easier. Try to focus on the true spirit of the season and create a special haunted house for children, or let them have a "scary" party with ghost stories, rubber spiders and the old game of "spaghetti intestines and grape eyes".

For the younger ones, a costume party with pumpkin painting and other activities is always fun. The important thing is that you run away from your own kind to avoid any trace of sweets.

- Overnight Trips

The first solitary sleepover can be challenging for you and the host parents. Children who are old enough for sleepovers and overnight trips usually begin to manage at least some of their diet and eating habits, which is helpful.

Spend some time with parents before the event to let them know what your child may need, and be available by phone to answer their questions.

Offer healthy snacks for the child to eat and provide nutritious food to cook.

- Food Conscious Children

It is important to teach your child the types of foods he is supposed to eat. Take the time to teach your child the comparative calorie content. This will help your child make better food choices.

It is best to teach her to read food labels early to help her become more aware of food.

- Nibble The Good Food.

Children are very vulnerable to snacks, so it would be difficult to take them away from them.

The only way to prevent childhood obesity is to allow them to snack on the right foods. Give them apples instead of a chocolate bar.

Remember that eating is a habit. If your children have been accustomed to a healthy diet from the beginning, they will grow up healthy and strong.

Indeed, the fight against childhood obesity is not a problem. It's just in the way parents teach their children the right things to eat.
How to help your child fight childhood obesity

• Childhood Obesity - Helping Your Child

A child who is overweight or obese is a child who should be considered to have a temporary illness. Obesity is dangerous for the child's health and has effects on his or her social life, self-esteem and self-confidence. When you decide to fight childhood obesity, you need to think about a plan and tactics that you will use to fight this disease.

The three main keys to losing weight and having a successful diet are regular physical activity .

A child who is overweight or obese is a child who should be considered to have a temporary illness. Obesity is dangerous for the child's health and has effects on his or her social life, self-esteem and self-confidence. When you decide to fight childhood obesity, you need to think about a plan and tactics that you will use to fight this disease.

The three main keys to losing weight and having a successful diet plan are regular physical activity, done on a set schedule and without exception. Physical activity encourages children to get better and hopefully will lead them to focus on activity rather than food or dieting discomforts.

The next key to fighting childhood obesity is of course a diet, the development of a diet plan should be done after consulting a nutrition professional who has all the tools and information about your child and his needs. By making a realistic plan that takes a lot of time, you will gradually adapt new eating habits, showing your child that there are different types of foods and making him/her aware of the things he/she eats and their effect on weight and body. It is very important to make the child aware of the effect of different foods, as this helps to clearly identify the cause-and-effect relationship with the child.

The last key to overcoming childhood obesity is as important and as natural as the first two, it is to slowly and progressively change the behavior of the child, and sometimes of the whole family, the new behavioral patterns can be treated as rules first, make sure you explain why it is not good to eat candy, and most importantly you need to make sure your child knows that every once in a while they are allowed to make an exception and have a piece of candy, do not remove and completely block the candy from their life as this usually has the opposite effect on children.

The behavior change is major and if it has an effect on all the other keys mentioned here, you should try to set some rules at the beginning, if you can have a family meeting and set those rules, it will be beneficial for everyone, making the children feel that they are setting those rules, You should encourage your children to set rules and follow them, when you start, you can also join in their activities to show them that they are not alone, and from time to time you can explain to them how important it is to follow the rules and the benefits that await them at the end of the road.

A technique I heard about some time ago uses imagination and positive thinking to encourage obese children to maintain a diet and physical activity program. The parents have a weekly interview with the child and review all the events of the past week, both good and bad, trying to explain what happened and why, and complimenting the child on his or her achievements. Once the events have been reviewed and the points have been clarified, the parent and child close their eyes and imagine what it will be like in a month or two, with more weight loss, better physical fitness and a daily routine, they talk about all the benefits of weight loss, such as better clothes, better feeling, more energy, social admiration, etc.

• Childhood Obesity - What Can Parents Do?

With an alarming increase in the number of overweight and obese children, governments are setting up programs to weigh and measure school children, but is this a useful strategy? And what can parents do to help their children control their weight?

As the government has become increasingly aware of the problem of childhood obesity, schools in the UK now plan to weigh and measure all children at the age of 4-5 years when they start elementary school and again at 10-11 years when they are about to start secondary school. This measure is already in use in the United States, but how effective is it?

There are arguments that children will be stigmatized and that this will increase bullying and the number of children with eating disorders in the future. In addition, many people feel that parents should be able to say that their child is overweight and that the money could be better spent by doing something to help change the situation.

As a parent, what can you do to help your children keep their weight under control?

It is important to be aware of children's feelings - if they are being harassed at school, parents need to ensure that they do not feel "caught" at home by harassing parents, which will only increase feelings of isolation and failure.

Parents can set a good example by providing healthy meals and not eating junk food themselves, but it is important to allow certain treats, as being too strict may cause friction and could be counterproductive. If the whole family learns to eat healthy and tries to cook new healthy recipes together, children will not feel isolated.

It is also important not to concentrate too much on food. Although it is an important part of life and cannot be avoided, it should not become the main topic of discussion within the family. If children are constantly reminded of their weight and what overeating can do to them, they may develop an unhealthy attitude towards food. So be sure to focus on other things, especially areas of life that are not stressful and that your child enjoys.

• Childhood Obesity

Childhood obesity is a medical condition found in young children. Children who suffer from this disorder generally have a weight that is disproportionate to their age and height. It is considered an epidemic in many countries and is common in the United States and the United Kingdom. Statistics show that one in three children living in the United States is considered overweight. A number of factors are responsible for the increase in childhood obesity in the United States. These three elements are genetics, nurture and marketing.

Research has shown that children born to obese parents are likely to become obese themselves. Although this is often due to excessive consumption of unhealthy foods, some believe that the disease may also be genetic. However, this research is currently ongoing and no concrete evidence has been found to prove this. It has been found that some children become obese because of the way their bodies grow. Another factor that many believe is responsible for childhood obesity is called "acquired".

Many children in both the U.S. and the U.K. are not getting enough exercise. Certain forms of technology such as computers, cell phones and video games have created an environment in which many children do not burn calories by being physically active. Energy that is not used can be stored in the body in the form of fat. It should be noted that it is not technology that is responsible for this, but the fact that parents do not ensure that their children are exercising sensibly. In the West, many children eat unhealthy amounts of fast food or junk food, which have become very popular. These foods tend to be high in saturated fats and are low in nutrients.

The third element that is often blamed for childhood obesity is marketing. In the United States and Great Britain, fast food companies are known to advertise their unhealthy foods to young children, and some parents have begun to blame them for the increase in childhood obesity. However, junk food and fast food companies often emphasize that it is not their responsibility to monitor the eating habits of those who consume their products. They often emphasize that it is the responsibility of parents to ensure that their children eat well.

A number of complications can be caused by childhood obesity. Children can develop dangerous conditions such as heart disease or diabetes, and some can also develop cancer. The number of these overweight children will remain the same once they become adults. Some of these children are humiliated by their peers, and may even be insulted by their own families. As a result, children who are obese are likely to suffer from mental disorders. The current debate is about who is responsible for this situation. While it is easy to blame junk food companies, parents ultimately have a responsibility to ensure that their children eat well and exercise.

• Childhood obesity in today's world

Childhood obesity rates are skyrocketing just as fast as adult statistics and it is a serious problem that needs to be addressed immediately! Most childhood obesity problems stem from the fact that children were taller when they were younger, so the problem would inevitably come back. It is so easy to gain weight in a world where most people respond to a good and appropriate meal with prepared dishes, and where parents think that food should be used as a reward for children who do something good, all they do is contribute to the biggest problem of civilization and condemn their child to a life of fat.

Childhood obesity has many drawbacks, both emotional and physical. When a child goes to school, he automatically becomes a target for school bullies, other children pick on him and he starts to get depressed and lose interest in school, when school should be the happiest time in a child's life! To prevent this from happening, steps should be taken to help your child lose weight.

Obesity also has serious physical drawbacks: the child will be the target of chronic diseases such as type 2 diabetes, heart disease, hypertension, bowel cancer and high cholesterol. These are only some of the most serious problems they will face, but other more general problems will include: daily activities will be hindered by their size, nice clothes will not fit, and general movements will be slow because all the extra weight puts pressure on their organs and muscles.

Most often, obesity can be prevented at an early age, but as children grow up and learn to make a difference, they need to watch what they eat and take care of their health. Regular exercise is recommended, but that doesn't mean that going to the gym, going out to play soccer or going to the park are all good things they can do to get rid of their excess weight. Parents also need to look at their lifestyle. Childhood obesity is due to parents not setting a good example and allowing their children to be significantly overweight.

All of these problems and anxiety can be avoided with a balanced diet and moderate physical activity Don't waste time trying to solve the problem once it has happened, save time before it happens and prevent the problem!

• Childhood Obesity - The Modern Health Dilemma

It can be seen in playgrounds, rollerblading tracks, swimming pools and classrooms. Obesity is a modern-day health dilemma for today's children, who are struggling with their weight like never before. It's a difficult problem to combat, as you want to make sure your children are getting enough nutrients in their diets. While some children can get rid of their obesity, others take it with them into their adult lives. Childhood obesity can...

It can be seen in playgrounds, skating rinks, swimming pools and classrooms. Obesity is a modern-day health dilemma for today's children, who are struggling with their weight like never before. It's a difficult problem to combat, as you want to make sure your children are getting enough nutrients in their diets. While some children can get rid of their obesity, others take it with them into their adult lives. Obesity in children can lead to feelings of fatigue, worthlessness and hopelessness. It can also put them at increased risk for diabetes and heart disease.

How big is the problem? The U.S. Institutes of Health have determined that over the past 30 years, the number of young people with weight problems has doubled. Interestingly, the problem affects children of all ages and ethnic groups.

Overweight children may not develop socially as quickly as their peers. They may become lonely and have difficulty making friends. They may feel that their weight is out of their control and may not know what to do to try to prevent weight gain. In essence, obese children can become our lost generation.

Parents of these children may not realize how much obesity is detrimental to their children's emotional health. They may view obesity as a passing phase and may not understand the psychological damage that obesity can cause. They may even ignore their children's concerns, hoping that the problem will simply go away.

The causes of childhood obesity can be complex. However, it appears that there are a few identifiable triggers. For example, many families are now eating on the run because of their many commitments. Parents may feel that they don't have time to prepare nutritious meals for their children, so they rely on fast food and sugary snacks to fill the gap. As a result, children end up on a diet high in fat and sugar, but with little nutritional value. According to the American Obesity Association, one-third of parents think their children's eating habits are worse than they were during their own childhood.

Inactivity is another major problem. Children watch more than one full day of television each week. This is in addition to the hours they spend on the computer. As a result, they don't play outside as much as children of previous generations. In addition, many children may feel that they can't play sports because of their weight. Feeling defeated before they even start, they miss out on physical activity opportunities.

It has been shown that children tend to be strongly influenced by advertising. Unfortunately, many advertisements promote foods that can be classified as unhealthy. Children crave what they see on television and in movies and may not realize the effects of these foods on their bodies.

Fortunately, childhood obesity can be successfully overcome. Here are some tips to help your child overcome a weight problem:

- Encourage your child to play sports or dance.

If your son or daughter is uncomfortable being part of a team, exercise with him or her. Take out a ball and make a few baskets or turn on the stereo and start dancing. You may be surprised that with a little encouragement, your child will get up and start moving.

- Remember to limit TV time.

Research clearly shows that time spent in front of the television is unproductive for children and teenagers. If your children spend less time watching TV, they may spend more time exercising.

- Banish junk food from your home.

With a little encouragement, children will get used to eating healthy snacks such as fruits and vegetables.

- Consult your child's pediatrician to see if he or she can recommend specific weight control strategies.

Childhood obesity is a problem, but it is not insurmountable. The more you take an interest in your child's diet and exercise, the more influence you will have on them. Over time, your child will learn the strategies needed to lead a healthy life.

• Explaining the Causes of Childhood Obesity

Many people believe that the cause of childhood obesity is due to overeating and laziness and to some extent they are right, but the main cause of childhood obesity is twofold. The DNA of the child and its parents. If the child's family members have struggled with weight gain for most of their lives, the child's genes will make them more likely to follow the same pattern, but this can be prevented by healthy eating and exercise, which is the case for parents .

Many people think that the cause of childhood obesity is due to overeating and laziness and to some extent they are right, but the main cause of childhood obesity is twofold. The DNA of the child and its parents. If the child's family members have struggled with weight gain for most of their lives, the child's genes will make them more likely to follow the same pattern, but this can be prevented by healthy eating and exercise, which is the case for parents. Children mimic their parents' behaviour, so if their parents eat healthy and lead an active life, the child is sure to follow, but in this day and age this is not the case, and as more and more adults go down the path of obesity, more and more children follow them and end up suffering the same fate as their parents, even though this could easily be avoided!

Parents have the most influence in their child's life, they have the power to show their child that overeating and lack of exercise are not acceptable in a young person's life and that it is the cause of obesity problems later in life. Obesity has terrible side effects and daily life can be very unpleasant. Simple tasks such as climbing stairs, taking a shower and other general things take more time and effort because of the extra weight. It's even worse for a child, they need to be active and have fun!

The causes of childhood obesity are not so serious that obesity is preventable! If you teach your children to lead an active and healthy life, there is no reason for them to become obese, even if their family is full of obese people! Obesity is a disease of cause and effect, it is caused by many things, including overeating, and its effects are horrible, complicating medical problems such as diabetes, high blood pressure and coronary heart disease! Childhood obesity is preventable, so let's try to avoid it, let's avoid it and let's help our children lead healthy and happy lives, without health problems or emotional setbacks!

• Avoiding Mental Trauma From Childhood Obesity

Children have greater energy needs as they are growing. Unlike adults, children are more prone to illness. When they consume more calories than they actually burn, the extra calories are stored in their bodies as fat. Childhood obesity is a major concern today. It is estimated that more than 15% of children in the UK are obese. Read the article and find out how to prevent childhood obesity.

Children have higher energy needs as they are growing. A nutritious diet is essential for their healthy development. Unlike adults, children are more prone to disease. When they consume more calories than they actually burn, the extra calories are stored in their bodies in the form of fat.

Childhood obesity is a major concern today. It has become a universal phenomenon. Overweight children tend to grow up obese. As a result, they develop a higher risk of hereditary diseases in the later stages of their lives. Obesity is the cause of many diseases such as high blood pressure, diabetes, hypertension, heart disease, etc. Health problems increase with increasing obesity.

An obese child is often confronted with psychological distress. Teasing and bullying about their appearance can affect their self-esteem and cause them to lose their self-confidence. This can lead to isolation and depression from an early age.

Children generally tend to be overweight if their parents are obese. But genetic factors are less important in determining childhood obesity. Today, most children are obese because of poor eating habits and lack of exercise. Foods high in calories, such as junk food, drinks and sweets, are fatty and cause obesity in children. Children spend many hours watching television. As a result, obesity is more prevalent in these children because they spend virtually no time on any physical activity.

Experts advise not to stress children to lose weight. Rather, they should be persuaded to maintain a healthy weight so that they gain it slowly and steadily as they grow older.

It is important to educate parents and adults about childhood obesity. They should try to instill healthy eating habits in their children. Fast foods such as hamburgers, pizza, macaroni, hot dogs, chocolates, cakes and potato chips should be avoided. Eat a healthy and nutritious diet that is fortified with protein and vitamins. Avoid fried foods. Try grilling or baking foods. A healthy breakfast of milk, whole wheat cookies and fruit is a good start to the day. Keep your children away from high sugar soft drinks. Replace them with fresh fruit juices and other sugar-free drinks.

Activities such as gardening, skipping rope and cycling can help prevent obesity. Encourage your children to walk to school or the market, instead of just jumping in the car. Motivate them to play games such as soccer, rugby, tennis, etc...

Studies also indicate that breastfeeding a baby may reduce his chances of becoming obese later in life.

A small lifestyle improvement can protect your children from childhood obesity.

• The Secret To The Solution To Obesity: How To Eat To Lose Fat?

I used to interview elite bodybuilders about their training and diet to make a living, and I did for years and years. A recurring theme that came up over and over again when we talked about diet and nutrition was how much food the best bodybuilders took away every day. These men were teaching their bodies how to manage increasing amounts of calories without becoming fat. In contrast, the typical obese person who eats one meal a day and adds body fat at the drop of a hat. I work with a team of obese people and have had great success using modified bodybuilding dietary tactics to help obese people lose body fat.

The first thing to do for obese people is to establish a multiple meal schedule. The obvious advantage of this strategy is that it divides daily calories into smaller pieces. I ask the obese person to eat every three hours, which is usually five meals a day. Then we insist that they clean up their food choices. Some foods are easily converted to body fat (sugary foods, artificial foods and saturated fats) and others are virtually impossible to convert to fat (lean protein, fibrous carbohydrates). The body's metabolism shifts into high gear to digest protein and fibre, creating what is called the thermogenic effect of food. Body temperature actually increases when the digestive system is faced with the daunting task of breaking down hard-to-digest protein and fibre.

Multiple meals allow the body to manage fewer calories at one time and repeated practice of eating 5 to 6 meals a day teaches the body to become skilled at digesting and distributing food. It is better to eat 3,000 "clean" calories a day spread over six 500-calorie daily meals than a 1,500-calorie fast food mega meal.

The results are astonishing when obese people adhere to this approach. I have a man who lost 40 pounds of body weight in 40 days while simultaneously adding 12 pounds of muscle. He started at 240 and yesterday he weighed 200, which is much more impressive because he didn't lose any muscle during the procedure, he added muscle. He wasn't an ex-jockey with muscle memory; he's a 48-year-old man with no experience in weight training.

Obese people who cut calories end up losing as much fat as muscle and end up being miniaturized versions of the old fats. This modified bodybuilder approach melts fat while adding muscle: the obese person eats more and, as a direct result, feels energetic and vibrant during the process. In contrast, the obese person feels deprived of calories, denied and continually on the verge of a frenzy. A person who eats healthy foods every three hours is much less likely to overeat and binge on his or her diet than a poor obese person who eats only 1200 calories a day. The calorie-hungry obese person has set his calorie ceiling so low that eating a chocolate bar or a bowl of ice cream causes him to gain five pounds in 24 hours.

The addition of functional muscles and the development of strength allows the obese person to become mobile and to climb steps, get up from a low chair and work their mass. Compare this to the person wreaking havoc on his or her already weakened body. Those who rely on deprivation to trigger weight loss weaken the immune system and continually contract colds and illnesses.

Those who live with 1000 to 1500 calories per day live in a stressful psychological world of denial. A person with a high metabolism who consumes 3,000 calories a day can absorb an occasional binge much better than a hungry person; I allow my parents to cheat once a week: it allows them to feel psychologically free. The interesting thing about the fraudulent meal (not the fraudulent day - the fraudulent meal) is that by "being good" the 6 7.8 of the time, the sweets, fat and junk they crave and could eat are rejected by the body and classically lead to diarrhea.

I am training five obese people with whom I currently work - one man and four women - and they all achieve equally spectacular results: they all lose unhealthy fats while building functional muscles and eating more than before the process began. This counter-intuitive approach - eating more to lose fat - has been ripped from the cookbook of bodybuilding champions and can be used very effectively by anyone who wants to lose fat while adding muscle.

• Obesity And Diabetes

Health is an important asset that requires appropriate care and supervision. A fit and well-proportioned body gives you confidence inside and out, while an obese physique makes you feel dull and pessimistic.

Health is a major asset that requires appropriate care and supervision. A fit and well-proportioned body gives you confidence inside and out, while an obese physique makes you feel dull and pessimistic. Obesity leads to other diseases and makes our lives uncomfortable and unpleasant. It also causes emotional suffering, which is one of the most painful aspects of obesity.

Obesity is not only a cosmetic problem. It is a health risk. An overweight person is twice as likely to die prematurely as an average person. In fact, obesity has been associated with several serious diseases such as diabetes and stroke.

An increase in weight of 11 to 18 pounds doubles the risk of developing type 2 diabetes compared to people who have not gained weight. Studies show that more than 80% of people with diabetes are overweight or obese. This may explain the newly coined word "diabetes", which means the close association between obesity and diabetes.

Type 2 diabetes, one of the most common diseases in obese people, reduces the body's ability to control blood sugar levels. It is a major cause of early death, heart disease, stroke and blindness. Overweight people are twice as likely to develop type 2 diabetes as people of normal weight. Type 2 diabetes is the most common form of diabetes. In type 2 diabetes, either the body does not make enough insulin or the cells ignore the insulin. Insulin is needed for the body to use sugar. Sugar is the basic fuel for the body's cells, and insulin carries blood sugar from the blood to the cells.

The chances of this happening can be reduced by losing weight and getting more exercise. If you have type 2 diabetes, losing weight and becoming more physically active can help you control your blood glucose levels. Increasing your physical activity can also help you reduce the amount of diabetes medication you take. Losing a little weight can also reduce your chances of developing heart disease or stroke and free you from a body condition.

Studies show that you can improve your health by losing only 10 to 20 pounds. Weight loss can reduce the risk of developing several fatal diseases such as heart disease, blood pressure, and blood cholesterol and triglyceride levels.

• Obesity: Enemy Of The Heart

Obesity is a problem that has reached epidemic levels around the world and has been growing rapidly among children and adolescents in particular.

According to the American Heart Association (PCA), one-third of children and adolescents and 66% of the adult population are overweight or obese. If this trend continues, our children's life expectancy will decrease, making them the first generation to live less than their parents.

Obesity in its simplest form is excess body fat. Body mass index (BMI) and waist circumference measurements are the most commonly used. BMI is the ratio of weight in kilograms to height in metres. Normal BMI is between 18 and 24.9 kg, m2. Overweight is any measurement between 25 and 29.9 kg, m2, and obesity a BMI greater than or equal to 30 kg, m2. Waist circumference should be <40 cm in men and <35 cm in women. Obesity is associated with the development of hypertension, stroke, coronary artery blockage, diabetes, heart failure and heart rhythm disorders. In youth, obesity is associated with the development of adult conditions such as hypertension, type 2 diabetes and cholesterol.

It is difficult to associate obesity with any one factor because it develops a complex relationship involving lifestyle, environment and genetics. However, there is a causal relationship between poor nutrition and unhealthy lifestyles. Sedentary lifestyles, produced by an active lifestyle, overexposure to television, computers and video games, and excessive calorie consumption, upset the balance needed to maintain a healthy weight.

Education is extremely important, especially from an early age, to establish good eating habits and healthy lifestyles.

To get the message out and educate youth about the importance of prevention, the American Heart Association created the Alliance for a Healthier Generation in collaboration with former President William Bill Clinton's foundation.

Obesity, along with other factors such as hypertension, diabetes, hyperlipidemia and smoking, is a crucial risk factor for the development of cardiovascular disease. However, unlike other factors, obesity (after smoking) is the most variable of all.

By developing or changing good eating habits and increasing physical activity, you can lead a healthier life.

• Obesity Surgery

Obesity is the scourge of the modern "fast food" world. Obesity surgery is an answer to all the "weight problems" an individual faces.

Obesity is the scourge of the modern world of fast food. Obesity surgery is an answer to all the "weight problems" an individual faces. In tune with the times, it is a quick response to a problem that might otherwise take years to resolve.

As the name suggests, obesity surgery is a surgical procedure that allows a person to lose weight. It is specifically for people who have tried almost everything to lose weight or who have tried to maintain their weight loss but have failed in all their attempts. Although obesity is relatively harmless compared to other diseases, it leads to long-term health problems and reduces a person's life expectancy. For these reasons, weight reduction is of paramount importance.

A person should ideally undergo obesity surgery if they are morbidly obese. Morbid obesity is a condition in which individuals have a body weight that is 50-100% greater than that measured by body mass index (BMI). BMI is calculated by considering a person's weight in relation to their height. In medical parlance, a BMI between 30 and 40 is considered obese and lying above 40 is considered morbid obesity.

Obesity sometimes manifests itself in cycles. A person can reduce their weight considerably and, in a short period of time, they can simply gain weight drastically. This is why new, improved and innovative weight reduction measures are being introduced, including obesity surgery. Obesity surgery is not as radical a measure as many people think. An invasive medical procedure carries a number of risks, as is the case with obesity surgery. However, there are many bariatric surgeons who are experts in this type of surgery. Associated with state-of-the-art hospitals and medical clinics, complications are largely minimized.

Many people see obesity surgery as a quick fix, but nothing could be further from the truth. It is a comprehensive procedure that also includes, among other things, high-quality support and services from other health professionals such as dietitians and psychologists. The treatment plan is established over a long period of time. The surgical procedure for obesity involves the placement of a gastric band in the upper part of the stomach. This helps limit the individual's food intake. To do this, laparoscopic surgery, also called keyhole surgery, is used. This gastric band or laparoscopic band is adjustable in nature and can be completely removed if necessary.

Post-operative care includes one night in hospital following the operation. It also includes regular consultations with health care professionals who will advise you on any subsequent lifestyle changes that a person may need to adapt to.

Summary :

The inherent goal of obesity surgery is that the patient is able to achieve his or her weight loss goal. When a person loses weight drastically, the elasticity of the skin is lost and is left behind. However, most experts offer their patients a full range of procedures that can correct all the problems associated with dramatic weight loss. With this article, we hope that a person suffering from obesity will be able to analyze and evaluate their options regarding the same

• **Obesity is an increasing health risk.**

Obesity is a health risk. It can lead to a multitude of diseases in the future. It is better to get out of obesity to stay away from future diseases. Changing eating habits and exercising are natural and inexpensive ways to treat obesity.

High blood pressure, joint pain, diabetes, hyperlipidemia, heart problems, paralysis, liver problems, menstrual abnormalities, breast cancer, female infertility, low libido, endometrial cancer, mental stress, blood circulation diseases such as arteriosclerosis, cholelithiasis, etc. These are some of the diseases that can cause obesity. The list seems endless. But before we know how to end obesity, we need to know "what is obesity?

Who is considered obese? A person with a BMI (body mass index) greater than 30 is considered obese. But how does one become obese? In theory, the causes of obesity are genetics, consumption of fatty foods, lack of physical activity, eating habits, laziness and endocrine problems.

What are the remedies available to get out of obesity?

Liposuction: this is a surgical procedure that consists of removing fat from the body by aspirating it with a needle.

Surgery: This procedure usually involves surgery to the stomach and intestine to reduce food intake.

Diet pills: Most diet pills are for short-term use only. These pills are only effective if used in combination with exercise and a controlled diet.

Fat burning pills: These are short term fat burning pills. But the main problem with these drugs is that the results are short term. Once the medication is stopped, the fat reappears.

Exercises: This is an ancient technique for reducing obesity. It is a natural process, so there are no side effects.

Controlled Diet Program: Like exercise, this is a natural process. Here, a limited amount of food is taken that controls the formation of fat in the body.

Acupressure and acupuncture: An ancient technique, but nothing concrete has yet been proven.

No matter what method is used to overcome obesity, there is no better method than natural methods such as exercise and a controlled diet program. And if a diet pill such as Phentermine, Adipex, Acomplia is introduced, the effects would be visible within a short period of time.

In addition to the physical aspects, obesity can also make you depressed, alienate you from the world, and cause you to abstain from social gatherings. If you're obese, it's time to take action. Whatever remedy you choose, you should always consult your doctor for advice on the remedy.

USEFUL LINKS

- [The ultra-effective intermittent fasting method for weight loss and long life](#)

- [The Guide to Obesity Surgery](#)

- [The laws of obesity](#)

- [The complete guide to fasting](#)

- [Overweight and Obesity](#)

- [Treating Obesity and Overweight](#)

ENJOY READING!

www.ingramcontent.com/pod-product-compliance
Lightning Source LLC
Chambersburg PA
CBHW071113220526
45467CB00004B/1853